No More Muffin Top

The Dead Bug's Guide to a Flatter Stomach
Specific and action-oriented

Helen Talbott

Table of contents

Disclaimer

Important Information:

This book, "No More Muffin Top: The Dead Bug's Guide to a Flatter Stomach," is intended for informational purposes only and is not a substitute for professional medical advice.

Health and Fitness:

While the Dead Bug exercise can be a valuable tool for strengthening your core and improving overall fitness, it is crucial to consult with a qualified healthcare professional before starting any new exercise program, especially if you have any existing medical conditions or injuries. The information provided in this book is not intended to diagnose, treat, or cure any medical condition.

Individual Results:

The results you achieve from using the information and exercises in this book will vary depending on various factors, including your individual fitness level, diet, and overall health. The author and publisher make no guarantees or warranties regarding the specific results you may achieve.

Safety and Liability:

It is your responsibility to ensure that you perform all exercises safely and with proper form. Neither the author nor the publisher are liable for any injuries or damages resulting from the use of the information or exercises in this book.

Disclaimer of Warranties:

The information provided in this book is offered "as is" without any warranties, express or implied. The author and publisher disclaim all warranties, including but not limited to implied warranties of merchantability and fitness for a particular purpose.

Limitation of Liability:

Under no circumstances will the author or publisher be liable for any direct, indirect, incidental, consequential, or special damages arising out of or in connection with the use of this book, even if the author or publisher has been advised of the possibility of such damages.

About the author

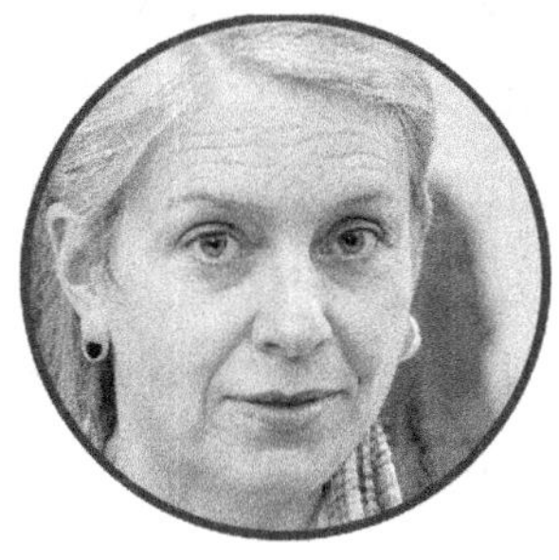

Welcome to the world of Helen Talbott, where fitness meets fun and results reign supreme! As a certified personal trainer and passionate advocate for mindful movement, I'm here to empower you to achieve your core goals and embrace a healthier, happier you.

My Mission:

My mission is simple: to guide you on your journey to a flatter stomach and a stronger, more confident you. Through my book, "No More Muffin Top: The Dead Bug's Guide to a Flatter Stomach," I unveil the power of the Dead Bug, a deceptively simple yet incredibly effective exercise. Forget restrictive diets and fad workouts; I believe in sustainable strategies and holistic approaches that nourish your body and mind.

My Passion:

My passion for fitness wasn't always there. Years ago, I struggled with body image issues and the pressure to conform to unrealistic beauty standards. But through mindful movement and self-acceptance, I discovered the transformative power of exercise. Now, I want to share that experience with you and help you rewrite your own fitness story.

What You'll Find on My Author Page:

- Sneak peeks into the book: Discover what awaits you within its pages—exciting Dead Bug variations, science-backed explanations, and motivational tips.
- Free resources and tips: Access exclusive articles, healthy recipes to jumpstart your journey.

Let's Connect:

Join me on this exciting journey towards a flatter stomach and a healthier you!

Remember, you are capable of achieving incredible things. Let's unleash the power within you, one Dead Bug at a time!

Introduction

No More Muffin Top: Conquer Your Core with the Dead Bug!

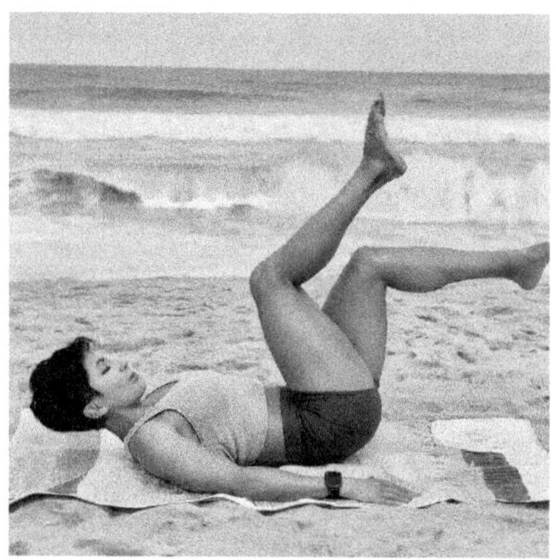

Are you tired of that stubborn bulge peeking over your waistband? Does the dreaded "muffin top" dampen your confidence and limit your clothing choices? If you've tried countless crunches and fad diets with little success, it's time to ditch the frustration and discover a powerful new weapon in your quest for a flatter stomach: the Dead Bug.

This unassuming exercise, with its funny-sounding name, packs a serious punch when it comes to core strength and definition. Forget endless sets of ineffective crunches that strain your neck and leave you sore. The Dead Bug targets your deep core muscles, the hidden heroes responsible for stability, posture, and that elusive flat tummy.

But this book is more than just exercises. It's your personalized roadmap to a sculpted core and a flatter stomach. We'll delve into the science behind the muffin top, debunk common myths about achieving flat abs, and equip you with the knowledge and tools to succeed.

Here's what you'll find inside:

- The Muffin Top Mystery Unveiled: Understand the root causes of this unwanted bulge and why traditional exercises often fall short.
- Meet Your Match: The Dead Bug Deconstructed: Discover why this simple

exercise is your secret weapon for core domination.

- Mastering the Bug: Learn the proper form and technique to maximize results and avoid injury.
- Unleashing Variations: Keep your workouts exciting and progressive with advanced Dead Bug variations and modifications.
- Crafting Your Conquest: Design personalized Dead Bug programs tailored to your fitness level and goals.
- Diet Demystified: Learn how to fuel your flat stomach journey with smart nutrition choices that complement your exercise routine.
- Beyond the Bug: Explore complementary exercises to sculpt your entire core and achieve total body transformation.
- Celebrating Success: Discover tools and tips to track your progress, stay motivated, and maintain your newfound flat stomach confidence.

This is not just another exercise book. It's a supportive guide, a cheerleader in your corner, and a testament to the power of small, targeted actions. With the Dead Bug as your ally, you'll banish the muffin top, unleash your inner core strength, and embrace a flatter, more confident you.

Are you ready to say goodbye to the muffin top and hello to a flatter, firmer stomach? Let's get started!

Chapter 1

The Culprit Revealed: Understanding What Causes Muffin Top

The muffin top, that unwelcome guest around your midsection, can cause frustration and self-consciousness. But before you declare war, understanding the "why" behind it can empower you to tackle it effectively. So, let's unveil the culprits behind the muffin top and explore the factors contributing to its presence.

Myth Busters: Debunking Common Misconceptions

Before we dig deeper, let's clear some air. Contrary to popular belief:

- Spot reduction is a myth: You can't target fat loss in specific areas like your stomach. Overall body fat reduction is key.

- Crunches alone won't do the trick: While crunches engage some core muscles, they often neglect deeper muscles crucial for core stability and a flatter stomach.
- Genetics alone aren't to blame: While genetics influence fat distribution, lifestyle choices play a major role in muffin top formation.

The Real Culprits: Unveiling the Enemies Within

So, what truly contributes to that unwanted bulge? Here are the key players:

1. Excess Calorie Intake: Consuming more calories than your body burns leads to overall weight gain, including around the midsection. It all boils down to energy balance.
2. Sugary Drinks and Processed Foods: These contribute to inflammation and

blood sugar spikes, promoting fat storage around the belly.

3. Sedentary Lifestyle: Lack of physical activity weakens core muscles and slows metabolism, making it easier for fat to accumulate around the midsection.

4. Stress: Chronic stress elevates cortisol levels, a hormone promoting fat storage in the abdominal area.

5. Hormonal Imbalances: Conditions like polycystic ovary syndrome (PCOS) can disrupt hormones, leading to abdominal fat accumulation.

Beyond the Obvious: Less Common Culprits

While the above are major contributors, don't overlook these potential influences:

- Sleep Deprivation: When sleep-deprived, your body produces more ghrelin, a hunger hormone, and less leptin, the satiety hormone, leading to increased calorie intake and potential weight gain.

- Certain Medications: Some medications, like corticosteroids, can cause side effects like weight gain and fat redistribution around the abdomen.
- Underlying Medical Conditions: In some cases, the muffin top might be a symptom of an underlying health condition like thyroid disorders or Cushing's syndrome.

Remember: Addressing the root cause is crucial for lasting results. This chapter equips you with the knowledge to identify the culprits behind your muffin top, paving the way for effective strategies in the following chapters.

Get ready to transform your understanding and take control of your core!

Chapter 2

Anatomy of a Flat Stomach: Unveiling the Muscles You Need to Target

Now that we've identified the enemies, let's shift our focus to the heroes: the muscles responsible for a sculpted core and a flatter stomach. Understanding their roles and how to target them effectively will be key to your success.

Beyond the Six-Pack: Unveiling the Core's True Powerhouse

Forget the "six-pack" obsession. While those muscles play a role, a flat stomach relies on a deeper layer of unsung heroes:

- Transversus Abdominis (TA): Often called the "internal corset," this deep muscle wraps around your core, providing stability and pulling your belly button inwards. Engaging the TA helps create a flatter appearance.

- Rectus Abdominis: Yes, the "six-pack" muscles do contribute to core stability and definition, but their true potential lies in working synergistically with the TA.
- Obliques: These muscles run along the sides of your torso, assisting with rotation and supporting your spine. Strong obliques create a balanced and sculpted core.
- Diaphragm: This dome-shaped muscle plays a crucial role in breathing and core stability. Proper breathing techniques can enhance core engagement and contribute to a flatter stomach.
- Pelvic Floor Muscles: Often overlooked, these muscles support your pelvic organs and contribute to core stability. Engaging them improves posture and can indirectly impact the appearance of your stomach.

Targeting the Right Muscles: Choosing the Wise Path

Now, knowing the players is only half the game. It's crucial to choose exercises that effectively target these muscles:

- Focus on compound exercises: Exercises that engage multiple muscle groups simultaneously, like planks, side planks, and dead bugs (of course!), offer efficient core activation.
- Don't neglect stability exercises: Exercises like dead bugs and bird-dogs challenge your core to stabilize your spine and pelvis, improving core strength and function.
- Mind-muscle connection is key: Pay close attention to the working muscles during each exercise. Feel the engagement in your TA, obliques, and diaphragm to ensure proper activation.
- Quality over quantity: Don't be tempted by endless crunches. Choose fewer,

well-executed exercises that target the right muscles with greater intensity.

Remember: A holistic approach is essential. While core exercises are crucial, remember to address potential culprits like diet, sleep, and stress for sustainable results.

By understanding the true anatomy of a flat stomach and targeting the right muscles, you'll unlock the full potential of your core and move closer to your goal!

Chapter 3

Debunking Myths: Exposing Fad Diets and Unrealistic Expectations

The quest for a flatter stomach is often paved with promises and pitfalls. Fad diets and unrealistic expectations can derail your progress and leave you feeling discouraged. In this chapter, we'll shed light on common myths and expose the truths you need to know for sustainable success.

Myth #1: Spot Reduction is Possible: You can't target fat loss in specific areas like your stomach. While certain exercises engage specific muscles, your body burns fat overall, not in isolated pockets. Fad diets promoting "belly-burning" foods are misleading and ineffective.

Myth #2: Crunches are the Answer: While crunches activate some superficial abdominal muscles, they often neglect deeper muscles crucial for core stability and a flatter stomach. Overreliance on crunches can strain your neck and lead to imbalances.

Myth #3: Detox Diets Cleanse Your System: The body has its own built-in detoxification system: the liver and kidneys. Fad detox diets often restrict essential nutrients and promote unrealistic claims, potentially harming your health instead of helping.

Myth #4: Quick Fixes Lead to Lasting Results: Fad diets promising rapid weight loss are unsustainable and unhealthy. Crash diets deprive your body of essential nutrients, disrupt metabolism, and often lead to weight regain once you return to your regular eating habits.

Myth #5: Perfection is Achievable: Aiming for an unrealistic "perfect" body can be detrimental to your mental and physical well-being. Embrace a healthy mindset that focuses on progress, self-love, and sustainable lifestyle changes, not just aesthetics.

Truth #1: Consistency is Key: Sustainable weight loss and a flatter stomach require consistent effort over time. Fad diets offer temporary fixes, but lasting results come from adopting healthy habits you can maintain long-term.

Truth #2: Balance is Your Best Friend: A balanced diet that includes fruits, vegetables, whole grains, lean protein, and healthy fats fuels your body and supports your fitness goals. Don't demonize entire food groups, as this leads to deprivation and cravings.

Truth #3: Exercise is Your Partner: Regular physical activity, including core-strengthening exercises like the Dead Bug, is crucial for burning calories, building muscle, and improving core stability, all contributing to a flatter stomach.

Truth #4: Progress, Not Perfection: Celebrate your victories, big and small. Focus on progress, not perfection, and acknowledge that there will be setbacks along the way. Be kind to yourself and stay motivated by your long-term goals.

Remember: By debunking myths and embracing realistic expectations, you set yourself up for sustainable success and a healthier, happier relationship with your body. This chapter empowers you to navigate the fitness landscape with clarity and make informed choices for your journey towards a flatter stomach.

Get ready to ditch the unrealistic promises and embrace a practical, sustainable approach to achieving your goals!

Chapter 4

Meet Your Match: Why the Dead Bug is the Ultimate Core Crusher

In the vast arsenal of core exercises, one often overlooked gem shines brightly: the Dead Bug. Don't let the funny name fool you; this exercise packs a serious punch when it comes to building core strength, stability, and yes, even contributing to a flatter stomach. So, why is the Dead Bug your ultimate core crusher? Let's delve into its secret superpowers:

Superpower #1: Core Activation from the Inside Out: Unlike crunches that focus on superficial muscles, the Dead Bug targets the deep core, specifically the Transversus Abdominis (TA). This "internal corset" muscle wraps around your core, pulling your belly button inwards and creating a flatter appearance. Dead Bug variations engage other core muscles like the obliques and rectus abdominis, too, for a well-rounded core workout.

Superpower #2: Stability is the Name of the Game: Traditional crunches neglect core stability, crucial for proper posture, injury prevention, and everyday activities like lifting groceries or playing sports. The Dead Bug challenges your core to stabilize your spine and pelvis, mimicking real-life movements and building functional core strength.

Superpower #3: Versatility - Your Personalized Core Playground: The Dead Bug's beauty lies in its adaptability. Start with the basic form and progress to advanced variations like single-leg dead bugs, arm raises, or resistance bands, keeping your workouts challenging and engaging. Whether you're a beginner or a fitness enthusiast, you can customize the Dead Bug to fit your fitness level and goals.

Superpower #4: A Gateway to Advanced Core Training: Mastering the Dead Bug lays the foundation for more advanced core exercises like planks, bird-dogs, and anti-rotation exercises. This solid foundation ensures you engage the right muscles effectively, maximizing your results and minimizing injury risk.

Superpower #5: More Than Just Abs: The Dead Bug benefits extend beyond aesthetics. Improved core strength translates to better posture, reduced back pain, enhanced athletic performance, and even improved balance and coordination. It's a holistic core workout with benefits that ripple throughout your entire body.

Remember: The Dead Bug's power lies not just in the exercise itself, but in how you implement it. Proper form, consistency, and gradual progression are key to unlocking its full potential.

Get ready to meet your match and experience the core-crushing power of the Dead Bug! In the next chapter, we'll delve into mastering the perfect form and unlocking endless variations to customize your core journey.

Chapter 5

Mastering the Bug: Step-by-Step Guide to Perfect Form and Maximum Engagement

Now that you've discovered the wonders of the Dead Bug, it's time to master its execution! This chapter will guide you through the perfect form, ensuring you reap its full benefits and avoid potential injuries. Remember, quality over quantity - a well-executed Dead Bug is worth more than countless crunches with compromised form.

Step 1: Prepare Your Battlefield (aka, the Floor)

- Find a clean, comfortable surface like a yoga mat or exercise mat.
- Lie on your back with your knees bent, feet flat on the floor, and hip-width apart.

- Press your lower back gently into the mat, ensuring a natural arch in your spine. Engage your core to stabilize your pelvis and avoid tilting it upwards.
- Extend your arms straight up towards the ceiling, palms facing each other.

Step 2: Initiate the Bug's Journey

- Inhale slowly and deeply, engaging your core as you do.
- Slowly extend one leg straight out, keeping it just above the ground. Simultaneously, lower the opposite arm towards the floor, reaching just underneath your shoulder blade, not directly behind your back.
- Maintain a neutral neck and spine throughout the movement. Focus on keeping your lower back pressed into the mat and avoid arching your back.
- Imagine your belly button pulling inwards as you engage your core muscles.

Step 3: Return and Repeat

- Exhale as you slowly bring the lowered arm back up towards the ceiling and the extended leg back to its starting position.
- Don't let your leg touch the ground or your arm fully reach the ceiling. Maintain controlled movement throughout.
- Repeat the movement on the other side, extending the opposite leg and lowering the other arm.

Pro Tips for Maximum Engagement:

- Breathe steadily and rhythmically throughout the exercise. Don't hold your breath.
- Focus on slow, controlled movements. Avoid jerky motions.
- Keep your core engaged throughout the entire movement, don't let it "relax" when your arm and leg return to the starting position.

- Imagine drawing your belly button inwards towards your spine to activate your Transversus Abdominis.
- Pay attention to your form and correct any imbalances or deviations from the neutral spine position.

Remember: Mastering the Dead Bug takes practice and patience. Start with slow, controlled movements and gradually increase repetitions and difficulty as your form improves. Don't hesitate to modify the exercise if needed to ensure proper form and avoid injury.

In the next chapter, we'll explore exciting variations to keep your Dead Bug workouts fresh and challenging, helping you conquer your core goals!

Chapter 6

Variations to Vanquish: Supercharge Your Routine with Progressions and Modifications

Now that you've mastered the foundational Dead Bug, it's time to unleash your inner core warrior with exciting variations! Remember, progression is key to keep your workouts challenging and avoid plateaus. This chapter equips you with a diverse arsenal of Dead Bug variations to conquer your core goals.

Level Up Your Dead Bug:

- Single-Leg Dead Bug: Increase difficulty by extending both arms overhead while lifting one leg straight up. Maintain core engagement and a neutral spine. Switch legs after each repetition.

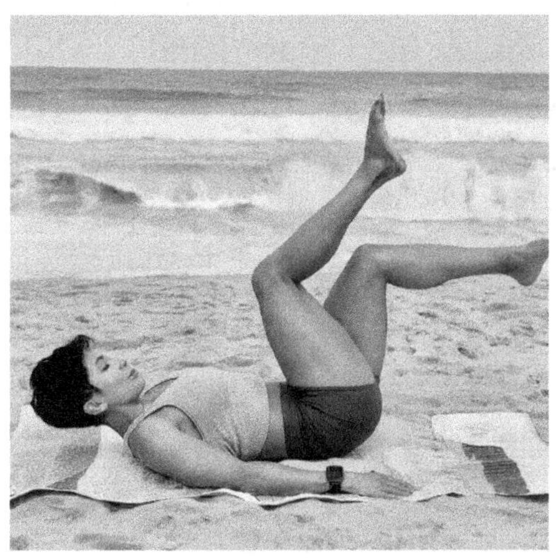

- Arm Raises: Add upper-body activation by raising one arm towards the ceiling while extending the opposite leg. Keep the other arm on the floor for support. Switch sides and repeat.

- Resistance Bands: Amp up the challenge by wrapping a resistance band around your ankles or feet. Feel the increased resistance as you extend your legs.

- Weighted Variations: For advanced exercisers, hold light dumbbells or medicine balls in your hands while performing the Dead Bug. Start with lighter weights and focus on maintaining proper form.

Conquering Challenges with Modifications:

- Reduced Range of Motion: If full leg extensions are initially challenging, keep your knees slightly bent throughout the movement. Gradually increase the range of motion as your strength improves.
- Isometric Holds: Hold the extended leg and arm position for a few seconds at the peak of the movement before returning to the starting position. This isometric hold increases core engagement and builds static strength.
- Assisted Dead Bug: Use a wall or chair for support if maintaining a straight back on the floor is difficult. Lean against the

wall or chair with your back and slowly perform the Dead Bug movements.

Customize Your Core Journey:

Remember, these variations are just a starting point! Get creative and explore different combinations of leg and arm movements, holding positions, and resistance levels to personalize your Dead Bug routine. Listen to your body, choose variations that suit your fitness level, and gradually increase difficulty as you progress.

Bonus Variations:

- Bird-Dog Dead Bug: Combine the Dead Bug with the bird-dog exercise for an advanced core-and-spine challenge. Extend one arm and opposite leg simultaneously, reaching forward with your arm and lifting your leg off the ground. Maintain a flat back and engaged core.

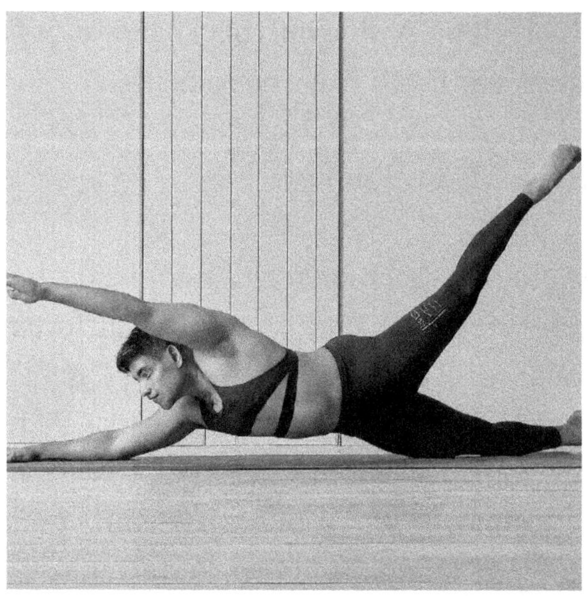

- Anti-Rotation Dead Bug: Hold a medicine ball or weight with both hands near your chest. Perform the Dead Bug movement while resisting any twisting of your torso. This variation enhances core stability and anti-rotational strength.

- Stability Ball Dead Bug: Introduce an unstable surface by performing the Dead Bug on a stability ball. This challenges your core to maintain balance and stabilize your spine.

Remember: Consistency is key. Aim for regular Dead Bug sessions, incorporating variations that keep your workouts engaging and effective. With dedication and the right strategies, you'll conquer your core goals and unlock a stronger, flatter stomach!

In the next chapter, we'll explore how to craft personalized Dead Bug programs tailored to your fitness level and goals, ensuring you maximize your results and stay motivated on your journey to a flatter stomach.

Chapter 7

Crafting Your Conquest: Personalized Dead Bug Programs for Different Fitness Levels

Now that you've mastered the Dead Bug form and explored its variations, it's time to personalize your core conquest! This chapter equips you with the tools to design Dead Bug programs tailored to your fitness level and goals, ensuring you maximize your progress and stay motivated on your journey to a flatter stomach.

Know Your Starting Point:

Before crafting your program, assess your current fitness level:

- Beginner: You're new to exercise or haven't exercised regularly in a while.

- Intermediate: You have some exercise experience and basic core strength.
- Advanced: You have regular exercise experience and are comfortable with challenging core exercises.

Define Your Goals:

What do you hope to achieve with Dead Bug training?

- Improve core strength and stability
- Reduce belly fat and achieve a flatter stomach
- Improve athletic performance
- Reduce back pain and improve posture

Build Your Program:

Here's a basic template to customize:

Frequency: Aim for 2-3 Dead Bug sessions per week with at least 48 hours of rest between sessions. Sets and repetitions:

- Beginners: Start with 2-3 sets of 8-12 repetitions per variation. Focus on proper form over quantity.
- Intermediate: Progress to 3-4 sets of 10-15 repetitions per variation. You can incorporate advanced variations.
- Advanced: Challenge yourself with 4-5 sets of 15-20 repetitions per variation. Explore more complex combinations and weighted variations.

Progression:

- Gradually increase repetitions, sets, or difficulty levels as you get stronger.
- Change tempos by performing slower, controlled movements or introducing short bursts of speed.
- Add new variations or equipment like resistance bands or stability balls.

Sample Programs:

Beginner:

- Warm-up: 5 minutes of light cardio (jumping jacks, jumping rope)
- Dead Bug: 2 sets of 10 repetitions per side (basic form)
- Bird-Dog Dead Bug: 2 sets of 8 repetitions per side
- Cool-down: 5 minutes of static stretches

Intermediate:

- Warm-up: 10 minutes of dynamic stretches (arm circles, leg swings)
- Dead Bug: 3 sets of 12 repetitions per side (single-leg variation)
- Arm Raise Dead Bug: 3 sets of 10 repetitions per side
- Anti-Rotation Dead Bug: 3 sets of 8 repetitions per side
- Cool-down: 5 minutes of foam rolling

Advanced:

- Warm-up: 15 minutes of dynamic stretches and mobility drills

- Weighted Dead Bug: 3 sets of 10 repetitions per side (2kg dumbbells)
- Stability Ball Dead Bug: 3 sets of 12 repetitions per side
- Combined Dead Bug: 3 sets of 8 repetitions per side (single-leg, arm raise, and hold for 3 seconds)
- Cool-down: 10 minutes of yoga or deep stretches

Remember: These are just examples. Adjust the program based on your individual needs and preferences. Don't hesitate to seek guidance from a certified trainer or physical therapist for personalized program design.

Embrace Consistency and Listen to Your Body:

Regular Dead Bug workouts are key to progress. However, listen to your body and take rest days when needed. Consistency and good form are more important than pushing yourself beyond your limits.

With dedication and a personalized Dead Bug program, you'll conquer your core goals and achieve the flatter stomach you desire! In the next chapter, we'll explore how to fuel your journey with smart nutrition choices, ensuring your efforts in the gym are complemented by a healthy diet.

Chapter 8

Diet Demystified: Fueling Your Flat Stomach Journey with Smart Nutrition Choices

The Dead Bug is your powerful core warrior, but even the mightiest warrior needs the right fuel. In this chapter, we'll demystify diet and equip you with smart nutrition choices to support your flat stomach journey, ensuring your efforts in the gym are amplified by the power of food.

Ditch the Fad Diets: Restrictive fad diets often promise quick fixes but leave you feeling deprived and ultimately unsustainable. Focus on building a balanced, healthy eating pattern that nourishes your body and fuels your workouts.

Focus on Whole Foods: Prioritize whole, unprocessed foods like fruits, vegetables, whole grains, lean protein, and healthy fats. These foods are packed with essential nutrients that your body needs for optimal health and performance.

Mindful Eating Matters: Develop a mindful relationship with food. Eat slowly, savor your meals, and listen to your body's hunger and fullness cues. Avoid emotional eating and mindless snacking.

Portion Control is Key: Pay attention to portion sizes. Use smaller plates, measure your food, and avoid overeating, even healthy foods.

Hydration is Your Hero: Water is essential for overall health and digestion. Aim for 8-10 glasses of water per day to stay hydrated and support your metabolism.

Sugar Smart Choices: Limit added sugars and sugary drinks. Opt for naturally sweet fruits and prioritize unsweetened beverages like water or unsweetened tea.

Fiber is Your Friend: Include plenty of fiber-rich foods like fruits, vegetables, whole grains, and legumes in your diet. Fiber keeps you feeling full longer, aids digestion, and can help regulate blood sugar levels.

Healthy Fats Don't Be Scared: Include healthy fats from sources like avocados, nuts, seeds, and olive oil in your diet. These fats support satiety, hormone balance, and nutrient absorption.

Protein Power: Lean protein sources like fish, chicken, beans, lentils, and tofu help build and repair muscle tissue, essential for a strong core and metabolism.

Don't Skip Meals: Skipping meals can disrupt your metabolism and lead to overeating later. Aim for regular meals and healthy snacks throughout the day to keep your energy levels stable and cravings at bay.

Read Food Labels: Become familiar with food labels and choose options with less added sugar, sodium, and unhealthy fats.

Plan and Prep: Planning your meals and snacks in advance and having healthy options readily available helps you make smart choices, especially when time is tight.

Seek Support: Don't hesitate to seek guidance from a registered dietitian or nutritionist for personalized dietary advice tailored to your specific needs and goals.

Remember: Building a healthy relationship with food is key to sustainable success. Enjoy your food, prioritize whole foods, and make mindful choices to fuel your body and support your flat stomach journey. In the next chapter, we'll explore how to integrate the Dead Bug into your overall fitness routine, maximizing its impact and helping you achieve your desired results.

creating your own personalized plan

Warm-up (5-10 minutes):

- Light cardio (jumping jacks, jumping rope, jogging)
- Dynamic stretches (arm circles, leg swings, torso twists)

Strength Training (20-30 minutes):

- Compound exercises that target multiple muscle groups:
    - Squats
    - Lunges
    - Push-ups or rows
    - Deadlifts
    - Overhead press
- Include the Dead Bug exercise! Start with basic variations and progress to more challenging ones as you get stronger.
- Aim for 2-3 sets of 8-15 repetitions per exercise, depending on your fitness level.

Core Work (10-15 minutes):

- Dead Bug variations (refer to Chapter 6 of your guide)
- Plank variations (high plank, side plank, bird-dog)
- Anti-rotation exercises (cable wood chops, medicine ball throws)

Cool-down (5-10 minutes):

- Static stretches (hold each stretch for 30-60 seconds)
- Foam rolling (optional)

Additional Tips:

- Gradually increase the intensity and duration of your workouts as you get stronger.
- Listen to your body and take rest days when needed.
- Consider incorporating other forms of exercise like cardio, yoga, or Pilates into

your routine for a well-rounded workout plan.

- Consult a certified personal trainer or physical therapist for personalized guidance and program design.

Sample Daily Workout Plan:

Warm-up:

- 5 minutes jumping jacks
- 5 minutes dynamic stretches

Strength Training:

- Squats: 3 sets of 10 repetitions
- Push-ups: 3 sets of 8 repetitions
- Deadlifts: 3 sets of 12 repetitions
- Overhead press: 3 sets of 10 repetitions
- Dead Bug (basic variation): 2 sets of 15 repetitions per side

Core Work:

- Plank: 3 sets of 30 seconds hold
- Side plank (each side): 3 sets of 30 seconds hold
- Single-leg Dead Bug: 2 sets of 12 repetitions per side

Cool-down:

- 5 minutes static stretches
- 5 minutes foam rolling

Remember: This is just a sample plan. Adjust it based on your own fitness level, goals, and preferences. Consistency and proper form are key to seeing results.

Chapter 9

Beyond the Bug: Complementary Exercises for a Sculpted Core and Total Body Transformation

The Dead Bug is your core-crushing warrior, but remember, building a strong, sculpted core requires a holistic approach. In this chapter, we'll explore complementary exercises that work synergistically with the Dead Bug, targeting different core muscles and contributing to a total body transformation.

Expanding Your Core Arsenal:

1. Compound Lifts: Don't underestimate the power of compound exercises like squats, lunges, rows, and overhead presses. These multi-joint movements engage your core muscles as stabilizers, indirectly strengthening them and contributing to overall core definition.

2. Anti-Rotation Exercises: Core stability goes beyond just your "six-pack." Exercises like cable wood chops, medicine ball throws, and Pallof presses challenge your core to resist rotational forces, building stability and improving athletic performance.

3. Planks and Variations: Planks are staples for a reason. They engage your entire core, including the deep muscles targeted by the Dead Bug. Explore plank variations like side planks, high planks, and anti-plank variations to keep your core challenged.

4. Bird-Dog: This dynamic exercise combines core activation with spinal mobility. Extend one arm and opposite leg simultaneously, reaching forward with your arm and lifting your leg off the ground.

5. Yoga and Pilates: Both yoga and Pilates incorporate core-strengthening exercises and poses that can complement your Dead Bug workouts. These practices also promote

flexibility and mobility, further enhancing your fitness journey.

6. Cardio: Don't neglect cardio! Regular cardio workouts improve overall fitness, burn calories, and contribute to a healthy body composition, indirectly impacting your core definition. Choose activities you enjoy, like running, swimming, or dancing.

Bonus Tip: Integrate these exercises into your existing workout routine or design dedicated core sessions, ensuring variety and keeping your training dynamic.

Remember: Consistency is key. Aim for regular exercise sessions, including Dead Bug variations and complementary exercises, and listen to your body. Gradually increase intensity and duration as you progress, and don't hesitate to seek guidance from a fitness professional for personalized plan design.

With dedication and a well-rounded workout plan, you'll sculpt a strong, defined core and achieve the total body transformation you desire! In the next chapter, we'll explore tools and tips to track your progress, stay motivated, and celebrate your successes on your journey to a flatter stomach and a healthier you.

Chapter 10

Tracking Your Triumph: Tools and Tips to Monitor Progress and Stay Motivated

Conquering your core goals requires dedication and perseverance. But how do you stay motivated and track your progress along the way? In this chapter, we'll explore tools and tips to celebrate your victories, big and small, and ensure you stay focused on achieving your desired results.

Monitoring Your Progress:

- Measurements: Take measurements of your waist, hips, and belly circumference at the beginning of your journey and track changes over time. Remember, muscle weighs more than fat, so focus on how your clothes fit and how you feel rather than just the numbers.

- Strength Gains: Track how many sets and repetitions you can perform of Dead Bug variations and other core exercises. Celebrate increases in strength and endurance.
- Progress Photos: Take photos of yourself at different stages of your journey. While focusing solely on appearance isn't ideal, progress photos can be a visual reminder of your hard work and achievements.
- Fitness Trackers and Apps: Utilize fitness trackers or apps to log your workouts, track calories burned, and monitor your overall activity levels. Seeing your progress quantified can be motivating.

Staying Motivated:

- Set SMART Goals: Specific, Measurable, Achievable, Relevant, and Time-bound goals provide direction and keep you focused. Break down large goals into smaller, manageable steps to celebrate milestones along the way.

- Find an Exercise Buddy: Working out with a friend or partner can increase accountability and make workouts more enjoyable.
- Reward Yourself: Celebrate non-scale victories with healthy rewards like a new workout outfit, a massage, or a fun activity.
- Mix It Up: Keep your workouts interesting by trying new Dead Bug variations, incorporating other core exercises, and exploring different workout styles.
- Visualize Success: Take a few minutes each day to visualize yourself achieving your goals. This positive self-talk can boost your motivation and confidence.
- Track Your Why: Remind yourself why you started this journey and what motivates you to keep going. Write it down and keep it somewhere visible to stay inspired.
- Embrace Setbacks: Everyone experiences setbacks. Don't get discouraged; view

them as learning opportunities and get back on track.
- Seek Support: Don't hesitate to seek guidance from a personal trainer, nutritionist, or therapist for personalized advice and support.

Remember: Progress takes time and dedication. Celebrate every small victory, stay focused on your goals, and don't give up! With the right tools and mindset, you'll track your triumph and achieve the flatter stomach and healthier you that you deserve.

Bonus Tip: Share your journey with others! Join online communities, find workout buddies, or even start a blog to inspire others and stay accountable yourself.

This concludes your guide to unlocking your core potential and achieving a flatter stomach! Remember, the Dead Bug is your powerful ally, but the journey to success requires a holistic approach. Embrace healthy habits, stay motivated, track your progress, and celebrate your victories. With dedication and the tools provided in this guide, you'll conquer your core goals and transform your body and mind!

Chapter 11

Conquering Challenges: Troubleshooting Common Mistakes and Overcoming Plateaus

Even the mightiest warriors face obstacles. On your journey to a flatter stomach, you might encounter challenges and plateaus. This chapter equips you with the knowledge to troubleshoot common mistakes and overcome roadblocks, ensuring your progress continues.

Common Mistakes and How to Fix Them:

1. Improper Form: Remember, quality over quantity! Ensure you master the Dead Bug form before progressing to variations. Don't sacrifice proper form for more repetitions. Seek guidance from a trainer or physical therapist if needed.

2. Not Engaging Your Core: Don't just go through the motions. Focus on feeling your core muscles working during each Dead Bug variation and other core exercises. Breathe properly and avoid holding your breath.

3. Neglecting Other Muscle Groups: While the Dead Bug is powerful, don't forget about other muscle groups! Incorporate compound exercises and full-body workouts for balanced development and improved athletic performance.

4. Unrealistic Expectations: Aim for sustainable progress, not overnight miracles. Celebrate small victories and focus on long-term goals. Comparing yourself to others can be disheartening, so stay focused on your own journey.

5. Skipping Meals or Rest: Rest and recovery are crucial for muscle growth and progress. Don't skip meals or rest days, as this can hinder your results.

6. Inconsistency: Consistency is key. Aim for regular workouts, even if they're shorter than planned. Skipping workouts frequently can derail your progress.

Overcoming Plateaus:

1. Increase Intensity: Once you comfortably perform your Dead Bug variations, challenge yourself with more advanced options, increased repetitions, or resistance bands. Gradually increase intensity to keep your body adapting and progressing.

2. Change Your Routine: Avoid workout boredom by switching up your Dead Bug variations, trying new core exercises, or exploring different workout styles like HIIT or circuit training. Keep your workouts fresh and challenging.

3. Seek Professional Guidance: A personal trainer or nutritionist can assess your form,

provide personalized recommendations, and help you adjust your program to overcome plateaus.

4. Monitor Your Diet: Are you fueling your body properly? Ensure you're consuming enough protein and other essential nutrients to support muscle growth and recovery. Consider consulting a registered dietitian for personalized dietary advice.

5. Get Enough Sleep: Lack of sleep can hinder muscle recovery and progress. Aim for 7-8 hours of quality sleep each night.

6. Stay Motivated: Remember your "why" and visualize your goals. Celebrate your achievements, no matter how small, and find ways to make your workouts enjoyable. Don't give up!

Remember: Challenges and plateaus are normal. By identifying mistakes, adjusting your approach, and staying motivated, you can overcome them and continue your journey towards a flatter stomach and a healthier you. Keep this chapter as a reference and don't hesitate to seek professional guidance when needed. Believe in yourself, stay focused, and conquer your core goals!

Chapter 12

Celebrating Success: Maintaining Your Flat Stomach and Embracing a Healthier Lifestyle

You've conquered your core challenges, achieved a flatter stomach, and unlocked a stronger, healthier you! But the journey doesn't end here. This chapter focuses on maintaining your success, integrating healthy habits into your lifestyle, and celebrating your ongoing transformation.

Sustainable Habits for Lasting Results:

- Regular Exercise: Aim for at least 30 minutes of moderate-intensity exercise most days of the week. Include Dead Bug variations, other core exercises, and activities you enjoy.

- Balanced Diet: Nourish your body with whole, unprocessed foods like fruits, vegetables, whole grains, lean protein, and healthy fats. Limit sugary drinks and processed foods.
- Mindful Eating: Savor your meals, listen to your body's hunger and fullness cues, and avoid emotional eating.
- Hydration: Drink plenty of water throughout the day to stay hydrated and support overall health.
- Quality Sleep: Aim for 7-8 hours of quality sleep each night to allow your body to recover and rebuild.
- Stress Management: Find healthy ways to manage stress, like yoga, meditation, or spending time in nature. Chronic stress can contribute to weight gain and hinder progress.
- Celebrate Non-Scale Victories: Focus on how you feel, your increased energy levels, and improved fitness instead of just the numbers on the scale.

- Make it Fun: Choose activities you enjoy to stay motivated and make healthy habits sustainable.
- Community and Support: Surround yourself with supportive people who encourage your healthy lifestyle choices. Consider joining fitness groups or finding an accountability partner.

Remember: Maintaining a healthy lifestyle is a journey, not a destination. There will be ups and downs, but focus on progress, not perfection. Forgive yourself for occasional setbacks and recommit to your goals.

Embrace the Benefits Beyond the Flat Stomach:

- Improved Overall Health: You're not just achieving a flatter stomach; you're building a stronger, healthier body, reducing your risk of chronic diseases, and boosting your energy levels.
- Increased Confidence: Feeling good in your own skin and knowing you're taking

care of your health translates to greater confidence and self-esteem.
- Sustainable Lifestyle: The habits you adopt now will benefit you for years to come, promoting long-term health and well-being.

Celebrate Your Journey:

- Acknowledge your hard work and dedication. You've accomplished something amazing!
- Share your success story with others to inspire them.
- Set new goals to keep yourself motivated and continue your journey towards a healthier, happier you.

Remember: You have the power to maintain your success and embrace a healthier lifestyle. By incorporating these tips and celebrating your journey, you'll continue to reap the benefits of your hard work and live a healthier, happier life!

Congratulations on reaching this milestone! This guide has equipped you with the knowledge and tools to achieve your core goals and transform your body and mind. Remember, the journey continues, and with dedication and the right mindset, you can maintain your success and live a healthier, happier life. Keep this guide as a reminder of your accomplishments and a source of inspiration as you move forward!

Delicious and Nutritious Meals to Support Your Flat Stomach Goals

Maintaining a flat stomach and a healthy lifestyle requires a balanced approach that combines regular exercise with a nutritious diet. While restrictive fad diets might promise quick fixes, they are often unsustainable and deprive your body of essential nutrients. The key lies in incorporating delicious and healthy meals into your routine that support your flat stomach goals without sacrificing taste or satisfaction.

Here are some recipe revamps and ideas to get you started:

Breakfast:

- Ditch the sugary cereals: Swap sugary cereals for a bowl of high-fiber options like rolled oats with berries and nuts, or

Greek yogurt with chia seeds and fruit. These options provide sustained energy and keep you feeling fuller for longer.

- Revamp your pancakes: Instead of using refined flour and unhealthy toppings, opt for whole-wheat pancakes made with banana or applesauce as a natural sweetener. Top them with fresh fruit, Greek yogurt, or nut butter for added protein and healthy fats.

Lunch:

- Skip the processed sandwiches: Ditch the pre-made sandwiches loaded with processed meats and unhealthy spreads. Opt for homemade whole-wheat bread sandwiches filled with lean protein like grilled chicken or fish, avocado, and fresh vegetables.
- Salad upgrade: Salads are a great lunch option, but be mindful of hidden calories in dressings and toppings. Make your own

salad dressing with olive oil, lemon juice, and spices, and choose lean protein sources like grilled chicken or tofu. Add healthy fats like avocado or nuts for a satisfying meal.

Dinner:

- Lighten up pasta dishes: Instead of heavy cream sauces and fatty meats, opt for whole-wheat pasta tossed with marinara sauce, grilled vegetables, and lean protein like shrimp or chickpeas.
- Baked is better: Instead of fried meats, try baking or grilling them for a healthier option. Pair them with roasted vegetables and quinoa or brown rice for a complete and nutritious meal.

Snacks:

- Ditch the chips and sugary treats: Swap unhealthy snacks for more nutritious options like fruits with nut butter, vegetable sticks with hummus, or air-popped popcorn. These snacks provide fiber, healthy fats, and essential nutrients to keep you feeling satisfied and energized.

Remember:

- These are just a few ideas to get you started. Feel free to experiment and find recipes that you enjoy and fit your preferences.
- Portion control is important, even with healthy meals. Use smaller plates and bowls to avoid overeating.
- Don't deprive yourself completely. Allow yourself occasional treats in moderation to maintain a healthy and sustainable lifestyle.
- Cooking at home allows you to control the ingredients and portion sizes, making it easier to achieve your flat stomach goals.

By incorporating these tips and recipe ideas into your routine, you can enjoy delicious and nutritious meals that support your flat stomach goals and overall well-being. Remember, healthy eating is not about deprivation, but about making smart choices that nourish your body and taste buds!

Conclusion

Congratulations on Your Journey!

Reaching this point signifies a remarkable achievement! You've conquered core challenges, unlocked a stronger, healthier you, and gained valuable knowledge about building and maintaining a flatter stomach. Remember, this isn't just about aesthetics; it's about embracing a healthier lifestyle that benefits your entire body and mind.

Key Takeaways:

- The Dead Bug is a powerful tool, but remember – a holistic approach is essential. Combine Dead Bug variations with other core exercises, compound movements, and cardio for a well-rounded workout routine.
- Consistency is key. Aim for regular exercise sessions, incorporating Dead Bug

variations and complementary exercises, to ensure steady progress.

- Listen to your body. Don't push yourself beyond your limits, take rest days when needed, and prioritize proper form over quantity.
- Fuel your body wisely. Embrace a balanced diet rich in whole foods, fruits, vegetables, lean protein, and healthy fats. Limit processed foods and sugary drinks.
- Celebrate your progress! Track your achievements, acknowledge your hard work, and focus on how you feel rather than just the numbers on the scale.
- Make it sustainable. Choose activities you enjoy, find a support system, and don't be afraid to seek professional guidance when needed.

Moving Forward:

- Use this guide as a reference and continue to explore new exercises, recipes, and healthy habits.

- Share your success story to inspire others and stay motivated on your journey.
- Set new goals to keep yourself challenged and continue progressing towards a healthier, happier you.

Remember, you have the power to maintain your success and embrace a healthy lifestyle. By incorporating the knowledge and tools gained here, and celebrating your journey every step of the way, you'll continue to reap the benefits of your hard work and live a life filled with well-being and joy.

Best of luck on your continued journey!

Dear Readers,

I'm reaching out to you today because I believe you might be interested in reviewing my new book, **No More Muffin Top The Dead Bug's Guide to a Flatter Stomach Specific and action-oriented**

This is a comprehensive guide to unlocking the power of the Dead Bug exercise, a simple yet effective move that can strengthen your core, improve your posture, and even contribute to a flatter stomach. Inside, you'll find:

- Step-by-step instructions for mastering the Dead Bug and its variations.
- Science-backed explanations of how the Dead Bug benefits your core and overall health.
- Advanced progressions and modifications to challenge yourself and keep your workouts fresh.
- Nutritional tips and complementary exercises to optimize your results.

- A motivating and supportive approach to achieving your core goals.

I believe this book would be a valuable resource for your audience, especially those looking to:

- Improve their core strength and stability.
- Reduce back pain and improve posture.
- Achieve a flatter stomach and a more toned physique.
- Find a fun and effective way to add core work to their workouts.

I would be honored if you would consider reviewing my book. I'm happy to provide you with a complimentary copy in your preferred format (e-book, physical copy, etc.). I'm also available to answer any questions you may have about the book or the Dead Bug exercise itself.

Thank you for your time and consideration. I look forward to hearing from you soon.

Sincerely,

Helen Talbott